Hope

Stem Cell Transplant through the Eyes of a Patient

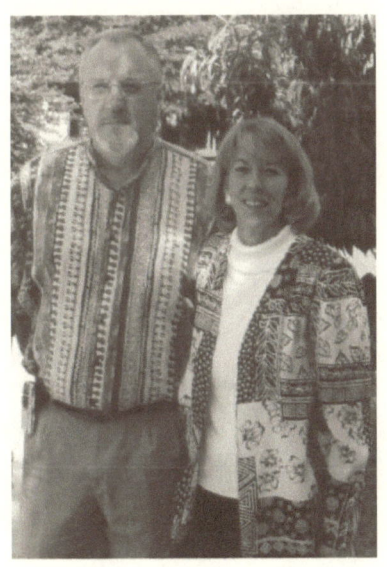

As lived by Harry Holmes II
As told by Sandra K. Holmes

TABLE OF CONTENTS

THANKS – to all that have stayed the course
with Harry and I through this entire journey.

We could not have endured if not for our children, Troy and Danielle. Thanks for becoming such great responsible adults at such a young age and taking care of us.

To our special friends that would go the extra mile for us no matter what.
Danny and Audrey Nolen
Mark and Anita Painter
RC and Tammy Austin
JC and Linda Nelson
And many more; too numerous to count

Thanks to our church family and many other church families for supporting us financially and with prayers through hard times.

Thanks to many of our co-workers that pitched in any way that they could, financially and with moral support.

Our primary care doctors, oncologists, specialists, and nurses have all been the best that we could ever wish for.

Thanks to Nick and Angela Holmes; what great kids. Thanks to the other family members that gave us support and loved us through our tests and trials. Love to Karen, Jerry, and family.

Hope

Sees the Invisible,
Feels the Intangible,
And
Achieves the Impossible

STEM CELL TRANSPLANT THROUGH THE EYES OF A PATIENT

Lived by: Harry Holmes (Patient)

Written by: Sandra K. Holmes (Spouse)

1

Auto and Allo Stem Cell Transplants in Simple Terms

First and foremost I think you should understand a stem cell transplant in simple terms.

When you hear a doctor talk about AUTO this stands for autologous and this is the use of your own stem cells. In order to collect your own stem cells, "mobilizing" chemotherapy is given to the patient and then Neupogen shots are started. When the blood cells start to recover from the chemotherapy, the stem cells are then plucked from an implanted catheter in the chest area using a leukopheresis machine. The cells are then frozen until they are needed for the transplant. Stem cells are located in the bone marrow and they are blood cells in the earliest stage. The bone marrow produces the stem cells into mature cells and then distributes them into the blood stream. Stem cells are sent into the blood stream as three different types of cells; red blood cells, which carry oxygen to the cells in the body, white blood cells, which fight infection in the body and platelets, which help the blood to clot and prevents bleeding. After the stem cells are collected, high dose chemotherapy (sometimes with total body irradiation) begins once more to the recipient. I personally call this the "Pacman" syndrome because the chemotherapy cannot tell the difference between good and bad cells. The result is many good cells die along with the bad ones. Then the patient is given a few days to rest. The stem cells are then intravenously fed back into the patient's system through the implanted catheter and the body is brought back to full strength with drugs, shots, and time. It takes two to four weeks for the body to actually accept the stem cells and function properly. Blood and platelet transfusions will become part of your daily or weekly regimen until the red and white blood cells and the clotting is accepted into the system.

When the doctor talks about ALLO this stands for allogeneic and means using a donor's stem cells. The allogeneic transplant is much harder to overcome as the stem cells, although from a matching donor, may still fight against the recipient's system. As Dr. Keung explained to us in simple terms, it is like having two persons living in the same room and they do not really get along well. A warden must be present to make sure they get along. Similarly, in the case of transplantation, an immune suppressive drug is used to prevent graft versus host disease (GVHD). The word 'graft' refers to the donor and 'host' to the recipient. These immune suppressive drugs may have to be taken for an extended period of time by the recipient to keep the two sets of stem cells in harmony. Unfortunately the drugs can be too harsh on other organs of the body, which causes many other complications including infection. The most common problems of GVHD include skin rash, diarrhea and jaundice (yellowing of the eyes and skin).

Both transplants are very serious and should be considered and discussed not only with your doctor but also with your family and caregivers. This takes a toll not only on the patient but also on the entire family that will be living the day-to-day journey. There are many patients that get in the express lane and the stem cell transplant goes very well. These patients begin the transplant, are admitted into the hospital and the full transplant is completed within four to eight weeks. They are then released to go home cancer free. The lucky ones remain in remission for years and must make quarterly, then six-month, and finally one-year visits for follow-up. Then there are others, such as my husband, who has experienced everything that any doctor could imagine. I guess you can say that the Bowman Gray Hematology and Oncology Team at the Winston Salem Baptist Hospital were *fortunate* to have Harry on their team. They were able to research many unknown symptoms and were able to diagnose many different infections. They have a better understanding of the mantle cell disease for future transplants, treatments, and cures because of Harry.

Please note: Hematopoietic stem cells are not the same as the controversial embryo and DNA stem cell research in process, which you may research on the Internet by keying cancer stem cell transplants controversy. Embryonic stem cells are completely different from hematopoietic (blood-forming) stem cells.

"We should not let our fears hold us back from pursuing our hopes."

(John F. Kennedy)

2

Early Detection is a Must

It was August 2000 and Harry Hugh Holmes II noticed a small dime size lump on the right side of his neck. Of course, with our busy lives, we put off many important decisions and checkups. Also in August 2000 we lived in North Carolina and our sister in Tennessee. We all took turns caring for our ailing 90- year old father, Harry Hugh Holmes I, who lived in Michigan. We were able to move dad to a nursing home in Michigan until he was able to travel, and then uprooted him from Michigan to Tennessee to an assisted living center near our sister. The family then had to empty his Michigan home of all of his personal belongings and put this home up for sale. We were also busy selling our small bagel and deli shop, so we were in the middle of a very busy time in our lives.

How many times do you hear the importance of early detection?   As the small dime size lump turned into a nickel, quarter, and then goiter size, we the family learned to stop bugging our husband, dad, brother, and friend that he must go to the doctor for a check up. He would tell us that he was so busy with his full time job and all of the extra stress that he just did not have the time. When he finally made the decision to make an appointment the real truth came out that Harry was just too afraid to go and hear the results that he was expecting. He knew that his body did not feel right in the last months and if he even had a small cut it would bleed profusely, but he failed to let any of us in on his fears. Read on and you will find out just why it is so important for early detection.

"Once you choose hope, anything is possible."

(Christopher Reeves)

3

Environmental Cancer

Another important question to ask yourself, is where does all of the cancer come from that is running so rampant through the American population? With the research that I have completed, not only with my husband's cancer but also my brother, sister, and father, who have all had some form of cancer, my understanding is that most of it comes from our entire country ignoring the abuse of our environment for way too long. Harry's cancer is most likely caused from working for a pesticide company 30 years ago when chemicals were much more potent and care was not taken to protect the skin or body. As the cancer lies dormant, in the body something (such as stress a big factor) triggers a reaction one day and it takes sprout, growing into a horrible killer. We were informed by Dr. Keung that the cancer rate for a 50-year-old male in America is one in every three will be diagnosed with some type of cancer in his lifetime. My family's cancer was also caused from pesticides.

> **"When the world whispers, "Give up,"**
> **Hope whispers, "Try it one more time."**
> **(Unknown)**

4

First Diagnosis – Small Cell Lymphocytic Lymphoma
First Round of Chemo

In February 2001, Harry went for his appointment with the Ear Nose and Throat specialist. A biopsy was preformed on the large lump on his neck. Dr Weiss guessed right away that it was cancer but told us not to be worried until the results came in. Harry was then referred to the oncologist and was diagnosed with small lymphocytic lymphoma. He was informed that he had a GOOD kind of cancer. My question was how can GOOD and cancer be in the same sentence? Immediately the oncologist scheduled Harry for 32 treatments of chemo. Harry took one week of chemo and then 2 weeks to recover while working his full time job as many patients do.

He did not lose his hair and took anti-nausea intravenous drip to keep the nausea under control. By the weekend he was very tired and worn down, so he would have to stay in bed to recoup for the grueling week ahead. He had one week of chemo with extreme nausea and, the second week was exhaustion and crumby feeling. By the third week he would be just back about back to normal and then it was time to "COME ON DOWN" and the torture would start all over again. He spent twenty-four weeks, or should we say six strenuous months, going through this treatment for the GOOD cancer. The rule of thumb for lymphocytic lymphoma is to receive your round of chemo and remission can last from months all the way to complete remission.

In the meantime, another lump showed up on Harry's right arm at the inside of his elbow joint. The lump to the human eye was the size of a golf ball on the outside surface of his arm. When the surgeon actually removed the tumor he informed us that it was the size of a baseball deep inside the arm. He said the veins had grotesquely grown around the tumor so blood could flow through his arm. The surgeon had seen cancerous cells many times in his practicing career and he called the oncologist immediately after surgery to set Harry up for radiation because he was positive it was cancer. The pathologist called and informed the surgeon that cancer was not indicated in the tests. The surgeon made them take a second test of a new biopsy and again, no cancer was found. The oncologist was just as surprised as the surgeon, but we sure were happy with the results.

"Courage is doing what you're afraid to do. There can be no courage unless you're scared."
(Eddie Rickenbacker)

5

First Christmas with the Big C
Pharmacy Rapport

At Christmas of the same year, 2001, pneumonia settled into Harry's lungs and he was placed on sulfa. Sulfa is used to treat bacterial infections and there are many patients that are highly allergic to this drug. At that moment we found out that Harry was one who was very seriously allergic to sulfa and it gave him a rash equivalent to a 1st degree burn. The inside of his mouth was like a piece of raw steak and the whites of his eyes looked like they had measles. He had to have aveeno baths just to be able to stand the unbearable itching and it took weeks just to start the healing of this awful reaction. You can bet that we have never used sulfa again. In fact, it is very important to have a good rapport with your pharmacist. Many times our pharmacist questioned the content of sulfa in the prescriptions given to Harry by his doctors. We have had as many as ten doctors assigned to Harry's case study at one given hospital stay. We have had oncologist, primary care doctor, pulmonary specialist, infectious disease specialist, pain neurologist, urologist, radiologist, cardiologist, orthopedic doctor, and the case study doctor. With that many doctors and specialists involved at one time our pharmacist would make sure that these prescriptions were never filled until thorough research and a call to the physician was completed. Our pharmacist was and still is a very important part of our daily life. Recently they found two drugs that Harry was on that contradicted each other and a decision had to be made which one was the most important for him to continue. Do not think you can treat this sickness as though you can go and buy your prescriptions off the mega pharmacy shelf. You do not know how important it is to have a professional critiquing your medication. We go to the small hometown pharmacy where the personal customer service is still available.

Harry ended up in the hospital for Christmas of 2001 and that was the beginning of a stressful, scary life endeavor for Harry and the immediate family. The oncologist rushed to begin a series of tests to include a PET scan, CAT scan, bone marrow biopsy, and a lumbar puncture. We were so fortunate to have an oncologist that had just moved to the Gaston area and her previous position was in cancer research. She joined the Gaston Hematology Oncology Group and we had the pleasure of being one of her first patients. We had only just begun our long journey and the next seven years made that first year seem like just a simple walk in the park.

"A journey of a thousand miles always begins with one step."

(Ancient Egyptian Proverb)

<u>6</u>

Explanation of Bone Marrow Biopsy
and Lumbar Puncture

Harry went to Gaston Oncology to have his
first bone marrow biopsy and lumbar puncture
in January of 2002. Just to let you know what a
bone marrow biopsy involves, numbing shots
are administered to the skin surface only
around the chosen area on the lower back on
the right and/or left side of the back. A hollow
needle is twisted approximately one inch deep
into the bone within a corkscrew looking
apparatus. The bone consists of the outer
covering called periosteum, the second layer
called hard cortex, and the spongy pink bone
marrow that lies deep inside the bone. The
marrow is the part of the bone that must be
extracted for lab testing to find the extent of
cancer within the patient's bone.

A lumbar puncture is even worse. The patient must lie in a fetal position the entire time of the procedure. Numbing shots are administered to the skin surface only, and this procedure is completed in the center and at the small of the lower back. A long larger needle must go perfectly straight into the spinal cord. When the needle is in the correct position a smaller needle slides inside the large needle and is used as a drip into a test tube (just like draining sap from a tree). My husband was not sedated for the procedure. We met a young man once who told us that he demanded sedation to do the procedure. When he found out that Harry did it without sedation, he said that he had to shake Harry's hand.

I was not allowed in the treatment room for the bone marrow biopsy or lumbar puncture. Neither Harry nor I knew what to expect the first time around with these tests. We were new to the procedures at that moment but little did we know how familiar we would become with them within the next few years. I had to wait in the hall just outside of the treatment room that he was in. I was extremely nervous. The physician's assistant that was performing the bone marrow biopsy was not experienced with the procedure. They were in the treatment room for an entire hour, which seemed like endless hours to me. The PA came running out of the room with frustration written all over his face and his entire demeanor spelled "Houston We Have a Problem". He ran past me in a blur and then my anxiety started rising. What should I do? I had no idea if there was blood involved. Could Harry bleed to death or was he already in cardiac arrest? Was I too late to save him? Could I have actually done anything to assist? After 15 minutes, I finally searched for a nurse to get some answers because the PA had not returned. When our oncologist finally arrived on the scene I felt like things would finally be under control, but she also had problems trying to complete the lumbar puncture. As time went on and we learned more about all of the procedures we came to understand why the lumbar puncture could not be completed as planned. After she tried for what seemed like hours the lumbar puncture had to be aborted. The bone marrow biopsy was not a success either. The corkscrew with the needle was not screwed deep enough into the bone and a good marrow sample was not available. We were sent home with a very heavy dose of pain medication to rest and only to wonder what the next step would be.

"Courage is not the lack of fear. It is acting in spite of it."

(Mark Twain)

7

Why Early Detection is Important

Here is the answer to why early detection is so important! The following week we were summoned to the oncologist office in our hometown. The news was not good. Harry had a new type of lymphoma that had only recently been recognized in the aggressive cancer family. In fact, he did not have the lymphocytic lymphoma but the very aggressive mantle cell lymphoma, which in 2002 only showed up in about 5% of cancer patients in the world. He was already in stage 4, the worst stage of cancer. Life was looking very grim. What if Harry would have went for a check up six months earlier? Would his cancer have been in an earlier stage? We can only wonder. If you read this book, please make sure you look for signs of early detection.

Many cancers do not have to be death threats any more with all of the new research and treatments that are offered today. Please talk to your family and friends and make them understand early detection is a necessity.

"Being deeply loved by someone gives you strength while loving someone deeply gives you courage."

(Lao Tzu)

8

New Diagnosis
Mantle Cell Lymphoma

Remember that we were introduced to our oncologist who was a research monger. With mantle cell being claimed as a new monster in the cancer field she was not going to be defeated by some unknown cells that could not be identified and conquered. Her nurse told us that our doctor stayed up until wee hours of the morning researching this new thing called mantle cell. Our doctor had worked with colleagues at Bowman Gray Oncology/Winston Salem Baptist Hospital during some of her research experiments. In January of 2002, she wanted to introduce us to Dr. Cruz's team but Dr. Cruz's team was involved in an experimental trial with a group of patients and did not have the time that we would need allocated for one patient. Dr. Cruz introduced our hometown oncologist to another wonderful oncologist specialist. This specialist was named Dr. Keung. He and his team just happened to be studying the more aggressive types of cancer at that particular time and were offering stem cell transplants as a research study. Mantle Cell, being one of the very newest cancer discoveries, was just what this team was looking for.

Harry was referred to the Bowman Gray Hematology and Oncology Group at Winston-Salem Baptist Hospital. We believed in our doctor and the specialists that we started out with and did not want to travel to another studying university in North Carolina.
What an experience our first visit to Bowman Gray ended up being in January 2002. We were introduced to Dr. Keung and he informed us that Harry was already in stage 4 and that

was the worst stage of cancer. He then asked us if we believed in a higher being, and we told him that we believe in God above. He said that he himself was only the assisting hands and if Harry was to live that was not within his realm but in a higher being's hands. He told us that he had a patient that has had cancer for 20 years and there is no reason that she is still living, but for some reason she is still on this earth. We knew we were in the right hands and already respected this man with Harry's life.

"Learning how to stand up is easy. Learning how to stand up after you've fallen down that is tough."
(F. Scott Fitzgerald)

<u>9</u>

Research Study Protocol – Tests

How do I begin to describe our first visit to
Winston-Salem Baptist Hospital? First, it had
to be determined if Harry could even be
considered as a candidate for the stem cell
transplant. What kind of transplant? Auto or
Allo? The exact strand had to be detected.
Would we fit into the research study trial? The
specialists had to consider the entire family
because it was a great trial for all involved. Let
me try to give the best account of the testing
program. We were first informed that this
hospital was a teaching hospital and we would
have a team of oncologist senior doctors on our
case plus a team of cancer specialist interns.
As the interns became more experienced they
would perform the ongoing procedures. We
agreed and signed forms to allow this protocol.

At this hospital I, the wife, was allowed and encouraged to stay for every procedure to give comfort to my husband the patient. Harry began his protocol by receiving yet another bone marrow biopsy. The biopsy was completed by a petite nurse practitioner who had to stand on a stepstool to get leverage in order to bear down on the tool that was screwed into the marrow of the bone. The lower back was cleansed, swabbed with betadine on both left and right sides, and covered with a sterile surgical coverlet. Shots were given to numb the surface area of the procedure locations. The apparatus was twisted through the hard outside bone layer, through the soft cortex, and finally into the pink bone marrow. As I watched this procedure, Harry would grimace with pain but said not one word. He was not sedated and had to lie very still. I watched as his toes would point straight down and than relax.

This happened many times until the procedure was complete. The bone marrow was extracted on both right and left sides and placed on glass slides. A lab technician assisted by collecting the specimens to complete pre-lab testing to make certain the biopsies were a success before releasing the patient.

Harry then had to get prepared for the lumbar puncture by first lying on his side in a fetal position. The senior doctor came in to do the lumbar puncture. The doctor examined the small of the back very carefully and searched the back for the hollow entry place at the canal. Then he placed a mark with an ink pen where the entry point should be. The area was also cleansed, swabbed with betadine, and covered with a steril surgical cover before starting the procedure. Shots again were given to numb the surface area of the entry location. It took at least 3 times of gentling sticking the outer needle into the canal, but Harry had a very stubborn path to his spinal cord because he had a curvature of the spine. Perspiration beaded up on the doctor's forehead and pain was written all over Harry's face. When the needle finally found the correct opening the doctor eased the four to six inch needle into the spinal cord opening. He placed the small needle inside the larger needle as a drip and the clear spinal fluid was caught in a test tube. A success. The doctor was as relieved as Harry when this procedure was completed. The curvature of the spine is what caused the previous lumbar puncture to be a failure at our oncologist office. He has had many very difficult lumbar punctures and Dr. Keung is the only one that we will let perform one without sedation.

The next test was the one that I would have run away from in a heartbeat. I will do the best to describe it so you can fully understand the extent of the gun and pinprick pain. They had to have a perfect pattern of the strain to know the exact cancer type and subtype in the back of Harry's neck where the cancer first appeared. Imagine looking at a tattoo gun as the needle shoots at a constant pace and extracts biopsy samples. No numbing shots were administered and this gun was placed on the beginning cancerous cell on the back of Harry's neck. The pathologist placed the aspiration gun on the neck and traveled in a perfect circle the size of a quarter as it continually pricked the skin and withdrew biopsy specimens. The pathologist completed the horrific test the first time and we had to wait until the results came back from the lab to find out that the pattern was not quite right. The next time they actually sent a mini lab to our treatment room so they could test the strain immediately after the next extraction was taken. Another practioner completed the same painful circular extraction test on his neck and when it was tested in the room on the portable lab it still was not a full perfect strain. The senior doctor came in and asked permission to try to do the extraction one more time for the strain type and Harry agreed. We were there for the best possible diagnosis and treatment so we wanted them to know exactly what they were fighting. They told Harry that a perfect strain is so hard to get and most patients would have refused a second time let alone a third. Our first day of tests was still not completed and it seemed like a full week had passed.

A nurse then came in and gave him a full clinical blood work up and we were released to go home but scheduled to return the next week for all of the test results and planning. Harry's pain threshold was really tested that day and the doctors could not believe the tolerance that he had. I told Dr. Keung that my husband was a much stronger person than I because I could not have even endured that first day of probing and prodding.   After a very tiring, trying and grueling day I remember food was not even considered, and we drove our 1-½ hour's home and fell into an exhausting sleep.

"It is not the size of the dog in the fight but the size of the fight in the dog."

(Unknown)

10

Results to the Protocol – Tests

We returned to Winston- Salem in just 5 short days for the test results and another apprehensive and exhilarating day since we had no idea what to expect. The doctor came into our treatment room and said that all of the tests were positive for mantle cell lymphoma. He sat down with us, drew pictures, and explained a stem cell transplant. He discussed using Harry's own stem cells versus a donor. The best decision for us was to use Harry's the first time and then years down the road if he needed another transplant his sister would be tested as a donor. We were told that we could go home and make the decision and then let them know if we would like to join their team of protocol. Our decision was made at that very moment. We were ready to continue wholeheartedly. Harry was not allowed to eat that morning and now we understood why. Dr Keung suspected that our answer would be yes so he had our nurse coordinator plan our next step for the process. Harry was sent to surgery to have a double port placed in his right upper chest. This port was called a Portacath. It would serve as input for intravenous fluids to transfer into the body, and as an output port to be used to draw blood from the body to alleviate needles constantly pricking him. After this was completed we were allowed to return to our hotel for the evening. Most of the research hospitals have a hotel in the area that will accommodate patients and family members for a very great discount cost. Harry was so tired that we grabbed a sandwich and returned to our room after yet another exhausting day.

The second day we went to the hospital again in the morning to find what our new adventure would be today. They would be ready to start the process the following Monday and if we were ready it would be "Houston It's A Go". This was now Friday and our adrenaline was pumping heavy with fear, apprehension, and excitement. We were able to go home only to return on Monday for admission.

"Take a chance! All life is a chance. The man who goes farthest is generally the one who is willing to do and dare."

(Dale Carnegie)

11

Accepted into Protocol

If this were a decision that you had to make, how important would a stem cell transplant be for you if the terrible word CANCER were branded into your life? With much research, great consideration, and the love that we had for each other and our children, we chose the path that we felt would be the best. Now we only had two days to prepare for the journey that would change our lives forever. We have four children and two were still at home so we had to leave our 15 year old and 18 year old at home to fend for themselves while we sought treatment for the betterment of our family's future. We were to be gone for four weeks and little did we know that our plan would be very different than the protocol that we had expected.

We returned to Winston-Salem on the first Monday morning in February as planned. We were admitted, tagged with the ever-popular bracelet, and made comfortable in my husband's new living quarters that were equivalent to a small hospital room. The spouse is again encouraged and allowed to stay the entire time in the room and there, of course, is the oh-so comfortable chair that makes into the oh- so comfortable bed. The nurses were great to help us get adjusted with the laundry facilities, making our way around the kitchen area and hospital, and teach us how to use the hospital café. We now were in our new home away from home and settled in for the blast off and count down. Of course anyone who knows us will tell you that we do not meet strangers so all acquaintances become like part of our extended family. The afternoon was spent completing blood tests and getting Harry set up in the system so all would run smoothly during his four-week stay. By Tuesday morning we were already a part of the Winston-Salem Baptist family including the nurses, nursing assistants, cleaning personnel and even the administrative personnel. The easy day was behind us.

The much anticipated Tuesday morning came and methatrexate, one of the strongest chemo's out there today, was intravenously fed into the catheter in Harry's chest. The oncologist team had Harry hooked to every kind of monitor imaginable. The team watched for any unexpected complications to the organs of the body such as the kidneys, bladder, lungs, heart, bowels, and the list goes on. By afternoon he was violently sick. I happened to be on the phone with my mother and I told her that the little bone shaped tray just was not cutting it and she had me get the wash basin that is stored in the cabinet in the hospital room. Sure enough that is how sick Harry was. For hours he filled the wash basin again and again. This was only the first day and we had at least four days of treatment ahead of us. What were we to think? Poor Harry could not even wake up without being sick to his stomach so the best thing for him to do was just sleep. I could not believe that this was the first day of treatment and it was already this cruel. I could not even imagine what to expect for the following weeks ahead. We finally made it through the longest first day of my life and settled in for a well-needed evening's rest. Harry was drugged up well so he could do nothing but sleep, thank goodness because Lord knows he needed it after the battle he had just fought.

Wednesday morning and the anticipation of the day was already high. The senior doctor and his team of interns were in the room bright and early to start yet another treacherous day. The methatrexate was administered again and the violent sickness began almost immediately. The team of doctors lingered around our hospital room consulting and comparing evaluations. Another day of the violent sickness and vomiting; then it was finally over again and the day was just another blur. The nurses ordered dinner for me so I could keep my strength through this ordeal and then after that I crashed with exhaustion. Harry was sedated again for the evening so that he could rest and recuperate.

Thursday morning came and our Pastor, Larry, drove 1 ½ hours to be with us on our third day of treatment. He came to give us moral support and I desperately needed it because I could not believe the affect this was having on my husband's body. The study team trooped in early and the methatrexate was pumped into

Harry's body yet one more day. The pastor and myself helped to comfort Harry as his violent sickness began and then the decision came from the senior doctor that the mission must to be aborted. Harry had gone through two full days and a small portion of the third day and his kidneys and bladder were in shut down mode. There was no way they could continue in this manner or Harry's system would shut down completely. Of course I was very glad to see the discontinuation of the chemo torture on Harry but also in the back of my mind was "No Stem Cell Transplant for Us". There were two sides to this coin and both sides seemed the evils (sickness beyond measure or no transplant). We were so afraid that we would not be able to have the transplant and Harry would not have the chance of a possible full life that we so hoped for. What a heartbreaking evening we experienced.

"Don't get discouraged; it is often the last key in the bunch that opens the lock."

(Unknown)

<u>12</u>

Change in Protocol

Friday morning came and the discussions began with the two senior doctors, Dr. Keung and Dr. Hurd. Harry had already received 32 chemo treatments the year before and his system was neither in the best possible health or strength. Most mantle cell transplant recipients start the transplant program from the first diagnosis and receive the methatrexate chemo while their body would be in much better health. They entered our hospital room with a new plan of attack if we were in agreement to their tactics. Remember, they were in research and needed to find out as much as possible about this cancer and what makes it tick. Also remember we were just patients with no other <u>HOPE</u> of survival. The research team needed to find the answers to help us and others just like us with this kind of aggressive cancer. So we were willing to go the extra mile with the "Men in White" for the HOPE and desperation of other patients that some day would be in this very situation. Lucky for us this was a team that did not like defeat and they sought revenge against 'mantle cell'. The decision was to send us back to our hometown oncologist and let Harry get CHOP (combination of four chemotherapy drugs) chemo treatments that are much less violent than methrotrexate chemo. It would take much longer to ready the body for the transplant but at least the body would be able to withstand the duration and severity of both the treatments and the auto stem cell transplant. How fortunate for us that this team was willing to try different methods instead of just following their protocol plan.

Harry's methotrexate trial study started the first week in February of 2002 as he received the horrible chemo then he had the following week to recuperate in the hospital. A game plan was put in place with our Winston-Salem team and Dr. Nicholson in Gastonia for his CHOP chemo to begin the third week of February. As Harry returned home and started his CHOP sessions he gained much of his strength back and bounced back to the fighting man that he used to be. Harry drove himself to chemo every day. He still had one week of chemo and then two weeks off. It was the same routine as the year before with chemo treatments; the first week he would be very nausea and sick, the second week very weak and puny, and the third week just getting some energy back and then they would ZAP him once more. He did lose his hair with this battle and I made him any kind of do-rag that he wanted to keep his head warm for the winter.

This regimen went on in Gastonia and we would visit our protocol team one day each month in March, April, May and June so they could keep a close count on all of Harry's vitals.

"Never confuse a single defeat with a final defeat."
(F. Scott Fitzgerald)

13

Immune Deficiency

Now you have to understand that Harry's immune system was very low and vulnerable after all of the chemo treatments because of the pacman syndrome (chemo kills all bad cells and many of the good cells). Going out in public for the immune deficient patient can be very hazardous to their health and they must be very careful and take many precautions such as latex gloves and special masks. The patient has a very low immune system and is very susceptible to all infections as they become neutropenic. A normal platelet count for a healthy person is from 150,000 to 300,000 cells. Many times Harry's would be as low as 12,000 and when it would go below that he would have to have a transfusion. Platelet transfusion is to prevent bleeding. When the white cell is low, the risk of infection is much higher. There are a couple of places that should especially be avoided by an immune deficient patient. One is a movie theatre because of all of the germs on the seats. The other is church because everyone wants to talk to you, give you a hug, and there are the children that are carriers of colds, flu, and germs. Let me offer you an example of the children being carriers of germs. Easter of the same year Harry wanted to go to church. He was so close to going with his special mask and latex gloves but he was feeling a little out of sorts that morning and decided not to go with us. I was a little hurt until I got to church and realized that he was not supposed to be there. My husband just loves kids and his special little buddy, Austin, always had his shirt un-tucked or tie crooked and my husband would straighten his clothes after Sunday school. This little boy was sitting in the pew just in front of us that day and during church he got up and went down the aisle vomiting as he went. The child had flu-like symptoms. If my husband would have been there he would have been so susceptible to the flu and I know he would have hugged little Austin.

So that was a very lucky day for Harry and I know that God forgave him for missing church that day.

In July we had a very new battle to fight. All of our children were home for the 4th of July and of course Harry wanted to attend church with the family. How excited we were as he wore his special duck looking face mask and latex gloves and came to church for the first time since January. When the doctors tell you the importance of staying at home for your safety they are not just talking to hear their own voices. They are telling you that because they know the dangers that we do not understand. Hopefully we can make our readers understand the importance of seclusion at the time of low immune deficiency. Shame on us for going against the immune system rules just to please the family.

"Hope is patience with the lamp lit."

(Tertullian)

14

Shingles

Three days after Harry attended church he started having very bad excruciating pain in his lower back. This pain then traveled down his left leg and into the bottom of his foot. He went to the hometown oncologist and there were no visible signs that showed up and she started running tests to see what the problem could be.

He already had an appointment in Winston-Salem to visit our specialty team the second week of July to have a Neostar port placed in the upper left side of his chest. This is a large port that would be used to pluck the stem cells from Harry's blood for use in his transplant. He went directly to out-patient surgery to have the port inserted.

While he was in surgery, I went to visit our nurses on the oncology floor. There I ran into Dr. Hurd one of the senior doctors and he inquired on Harry's well being. I explained to him that Harry was in such pain with his left leg and foot that he had actually discussed with me that he would like to consider having his left leg removed because of the excruciating pain. As Harry was not a person to complain about pain this was a very serious request on his part. Dr. Hurd immediately knew the problem without even an examination and called the team to place Harry in quarantine. The doctor guessed at the diagnosis and was correct that Harry had shingles. A gentleman at our church had been diagnosed with shingles the week before and was a carrier of the infection. If Harry would have stayed home from church as he was advised he could have saved himself a lot of pain and suffering.

Harry was quarantined to a hospital room with shingles that traveled from the nerve endings in his lower back down his left leg and then into his left foot which caused neuropathy. Neuropathy caused the toes of his left foot to drag and then he would fall because he was not able to walk properly. This condition is also called 'dropped foot'. He was measured for a brace for his 'dropped foot' and was told that he would never be able to walk again without the brace. He did prove them wrong in this sense as he began rehabilitation and within one year he was able to remove the brace and walk again without assistance.

With his week immune system the shingles continued to travel through his system. With constant chest x-rays they monitored the damage that the shingle trail was leaving in its path. There were lesions on his lungs and that caused his lungs to be filled with fluids and this was caused by bacterial pneumonia that he contracted at the same time. This was one of the most painful experiences I have seen anyone go through in a lifetime. The fluids would continue to fill the lungs and as he would sit up his chest sounded like a 55-gallon drum with the sloshing of the fluids. There were times that neither the doctors nor I thought that Harry would make it out of the hospital alive with this serious illness. He was in the hospital for three weeks. At the end of the third week Harry surprised everyone and was released to go home.

"Hope is faith holding out its hand in the dark."

(George Iles)

15

More Complications
Fungus and Bronchiectasis

Harry's release from the hospital was only a short one. In just three short days he was rushed back to Winston-Salem Baptist Hospital with more complications. This ran us into August of 2002 and we were worried because we were behind on chemo treatments. We lived in a moldy apartment at the time and with the shingles and bacterial pneumonia that Harry had experienced along came a new unknown. He was placed back in the hospital and extensive tests were run to find out that bacterial infection was the diagnosis. This was treated for days and Harry was just getting sicker by the day. He was very close to death. I mentioned the mold in our apartment and also that Harry's little dog had just been treated for a fungal infection. Dr. Keung tested Harry for fungal infection and it kept showing up as bacterial. Since Harry and I were so adamant about the fungus in our apartment they treated him for fungal infection. The infection soon started clearing up. The doctors found out that with all the tests that they ran on Harry his results would be just opposite of the diagnosis. Wouldn't you know he had to be just another puzzle for them to solve?

In the meantime, his fungal infection transformed into bronchiectasis and the lung specialists were called in to help solve yet another complication. With each of the new symptoms would come a new test and diagnosis. The tests were interesting as they would take a sputum culture or a biopsy of the lung or mucus from the bronchial tube and then let the culture grow in a petri dish until the correct diagnosis could be made and treated. Then with Harry's backward system the medication prescribed may not have been the correct one after all. Harry had so many complications already and the stem cell transplant had not even begun as of yet. He was at a very weak state now and his chemo treatments had to be stopped during the five weeks that he was admitted in the hospital for shingles, fungal infection and bronchiectasis. Many times he was close to death's door.

"Life shrinks or expands in proportion to
one's courage."
(Anis Nin)

16

Transplant Decision Must be Made

The transplant was getting closer and he had to return to Winston-Salem Baptist Hospital twice a month during August, September, and October. He had three bone marrow biopsies during the nine months of pre transplant visits. Wouldn't it be interesting to see an x-ray of Harry's lower back with all of the bone marrow biopsies and lumbar punctures that he had received and with many more to come? I am sure that it would be full of holes. Remember he was on the regimen of CHOP chemo treatments and that, in my opinion, was more than I could have handled. He endured so much pain and tolerated it so well. He is a hero in my book just for putting up with the pain and living through all that he had so far on this journey and we were not even in the stem cell transplant stage yet.

Harry was in no position to complete his CHOP chemo sessions and the team knew that if the transplant were not completed soon there would be no chance to continue with the plan because he was getting weaker, not stronger.

"Trust the still small voice that says,
This might work and I'll try it."
(Diane Mariechild)

<u>17</u>

Auto Stem Cell Transplant Begins

On October 21, 2002, Harry was admitted into
Bowman Gray Oncology, Winston-Salem
Baptist Hospital to begin his auto stem cell
transplant. What a momentous day for Harry.
He had worked so hard and gone through so
much for this moment. Of course do not think
that Harry was going to get a free ride without
a lot of hard work for this transplant. He gave
the doctors a run for their money and he had
many terrible days ahead of him.

The first day was spent settling into our small
but cozy hospital room. Harry received all of
his blood tests and was entered into the system
to make sure the next four weeks were a
smooth stay.

On the same day chemo was injected into the spinal cord to eliminate any remaining cancer cells. Surprisingly, there is a brain barrier so chemo is blocked from the brain, so it remains in the spinal cord to do its job of eating bad cells. Since the regular chemotherapy given through the veins cannot reach the brain and spinal cord due to the presence of the blood brain barrier, special "intrathecal" chemotherapy has to be given directly to the spinal region through a lumbar puncture in order to kill the lymphoma cells that may have hidden in the brain and spinal cord. The chemotherapy given in the spinal region eventually circulates to the whole brain within the craniospinal fluid.

The second day would begin yet another adventurous journey for the Holmes family and the protocol team. One million stem cells were to be plucked from Harry's Neostar catheter. Two full days of eight hours each were spent collecting peripheral blood stem cells (PBSC). He would receive shots to build the stem cells so they could be collected for harvesting. Many times the patient goes to the pheresis department for collection. The pheresis nurse would bring the collection machine right to the hospital room and sterilize every thing and hook the tubing into Harry's Neostar catheter in his left upper chest. She would stay right by his bedside to make sure there were no complications. Let me try to describe the stem cell collection machine to the best of my ability. Clear plastic tubing is attached to the catheter port that has been implanted in the patient's chest months earlier. Blood is drawn out of the body and it flows through this plastic tubing that runs on a large complicated board in the shape of a large curvy snake. This machine has many dials and electrodes to divide the new cells from the mature cells as the blood is collected from the body. It has a two-gallon size plastic bag as the dumpsite on the other end of the board. All stem cells (blood in the earliest stage) as they are referred to are collected in the large plastic bag and the mature blood is sent back into the body through the input of the Neostar catheter. This machine is a very complicated looking contraption.

Of course you probably have guessed it. Harry had to be the one patient in a million that gave them every possibility of thorough research. On the third day Dr. Keung came to Harry's hospital room and told us the terrible news. Out of one million stem cells, they were only able to pluck one hundred thousand stem cells from Harry's system. Due to his entire sickness, stem cells (new blood) were not being reproduced in his body. The real scare came because I heard of this problem with another patient a few months earlier and she was informed that they could not continue the process and she would have to return home without the transplant. We were stricken of all this hard work, sickness and extra complications and there was now no <u>HOPE</u> for us once again.

In the meantime, Harry's Neostar port became infected with a staph infection. He had to be taken into surgery to have the port removed. He would tell you that it was not a fun task at hand to have a port removed that had become infected. Of course, once again, they did not sedate him as they started to remove the implanted chest port. A smaller technician tugged and pulled and could not remove the port. He left Harry's side and returned with a big guy and it literally took the man placing his knee on the chest area to pull the infected port out. Harry said it was like a mule kicking him

in the chest to have that thing removed.
Cancer patients should be very careful with
infections.

"Courage doesn't always roar. Sometimes
courage is the little voice at the end of the day
that says.....I'll try again tomorrow."
(Mary Anne Radmacher – Hershey)

<u>18</u>

Change in Plan

Dr. Keung was very serious about this transplant, and had an idea that he would like to try if we were willing to listen. He and another senior surgeon would sedate Harry and they would make multiple aspirations through small skin incisions made on both sides of Harry's hip bones, and remove enough of his bone marrow to use for his transplant. Harry would then be receiving a stem cell and bone marrow transplant by using his own cells and marrow. After the removal they would have to run this marrow through the filter to remove any bone chips. The cells and marrow would then be harvested and frozen for the transplant. They gave Harry a 50/50 chance of making it and the doctor was going to let us go home to make the decision, but of course we knew our decision during the discussion. We were in the hands of an awesome oncologist team and we had full trust and respect in them. Once again we said, "Let's Go For It". Harry had a 50/50 chance of making it through this stem cell transplant. After all of the miracles he had already been through, what is one more try? What did he have to loose?

The third day in the hospital began early am with Harry being wheeled into surgery. Fourteen incisions were made in Harry's lower back and the bone marrow was removed from his back for the transplant by the two surgeons. He was kept sedated for the remaining of the day and for the entire fourth day. The days ahead were just a blur to Harry.

The fourth and fifth days Harry received high dose Cyclophospamide Chemo to make sure that the bad cells were killed in their entirety.

These were two more terrible days in the eyes of the caregiver. The sixth day is a day of absolute rest for the body, so they kept him sedated and he slept as restful as a small baby. The seventh, eighth, ninth, and tenth days were spent receiving total body radiation twice daily. Harry said that he had to set on a stool in a fetal position for 45 minutes twice a day. He remembered how hard it was to sit there and keep control of his muscles so he would not fall off from the freestanding stool or move for fear that the radiation would shoot into the incorrect area. In many ways radiation is worse than chemo as it exhausts all energy that the body or muscles have. Fortunately the rays did not burn his skin and that was a great factor in this situation.

Another great thing about our medical journey is neither Harry nor I were subject to adverse change. We have had so many twists and turns in our adventure and that made it all the more interesting and exciting to live. By this time in the game we had already experienced an awesome journey and we still had miles to go.

"Do not go where the path may lead instead go where there is no path and leave a trail."
(Ralph Waldo Emerson)

<u>19</u>

Days of Wonderment

Harry could not stand light or even the sound
of television or music in his hospital room.
Fresh fruit, vegetables, live-plants, nor visitors
were allowed in his room. I spent the next five
days reading in the bathroom of his room so I
would be there when he needed someone. He
was in total and complete care of others. He
was given intravenous fluid, had to wear
diapers, and did not remember anything that
happened over the next five days.

Then like magic, Harry woke up and was
feeling pretty perky. I called him Rip-Van-
Winkle. I recall he even ate a small portion of
solid food that day. His temperature, heart,
oxygen level, and blood pressure were
monitored and all seemed at a safe and steady

level. On the morning of Friday, November 1, 2002 the process was set up and the stem cell transplant would begin. This would be considered Harry's new birthday as he was literally at death and brought back to life with his own purged cells. He would have to receive all of his baby shots again. He would have to receive both flu and pneumonia shots each year for the remainder of his life. .

"Hope is the word which God has written on the brow of every man."

(Victor Hugo)

<u>20</u>

The Actual Stem Cell Process Day

Where do we begin with this long and exciting day? First the room was emptied of everything except Harry's hospital bed. This was a precautionary measure in case they had to bring specialist teams in from cardiac or pulmonary.   In the early morning the stem cells were brought from the lab freezer and placed in the room on the sterile table to begin the thaw. They were in two large hypodermic needle tubes approximately 2 inches in diameter and six inches in length. They reminded me of a frosting tube with a large T-shaped handle to press. The cells looked just like a thick liver paste with a very deep red color.

As they were prepping Harry for the
transplant the team was describing some
things that would happen. As the door of the
hospital room is closed the entire hallway
begins to smell like creamed corn. Anytime a
transplant was being performed I could tell by
the smell of creamed corn in the hallway. Most
recipients vomit during the transplant because
it is injected into the tube in the chest and must
pass through the veins and they can taste it
and it also gathers in their throat as it thins out
in the blood stream. The team brings in
lollipops for the patient so it takes the mind
away from the matter at hand. Boy, Harry was
looking forward to another fun day of that.
They continued to ready the room and I was
allowed to stay for the full process and even sit
upon the bed. I was really not looking forward
to another sick day either, but I was there for
the duration. One of the soon to graduate
interns actually performed the procedure and

it was her suggestion to let Harry assist. That was a perfect idea and I hope they have continued with that because the day was very amazing.

The stem cell transplant began by giving Harry his lollipop. He was so interested in his assisting job that he did not even bother with the candy. The female intern explained Harry's job to him. He was so funny and so intent on doing this right. Let me try to describe this process so you can actually picture it in your mind. The stem cells must be mixed with saline solution to thin the mixture out so it can be accepted into the bone marrow. Plastic tubing is attached to the catheter in the chest and following down the tubing there is a T-tube connection. On one side of the T is the needle filled with stem cells/bone marrow and on the other side of the T is the bag of solution. This would be intravenously fed into the body.

On one side of the t-connection Harry had a small dial that looked like the on/off switch on a nite-lite and on the other side of the t-connection a large tube of cells was attached. Harry would have to roll the switch on and the doctor would push on the large needle to pump stem cells and bone marrow into his port. As he turned the switch on the solution would mix with the thick substance so it could then enter into the port. He would then turn his switch off and she would stop pushing on her needle. The doctor and Harry continued what seemed like forever and Harry was so serious about his job that he never once vomited. All he could ask was "How am I doing Doc?" The doctor was so tired from pumping the cells because they were so thick and you could just see her hands shake with fatigue. I knew that being a small female intern she had to complete the transplant, as she must be made ready to continue on in life as an oncologist specialist. I believe that with Harry's mind on something besides the process it was a great help to all involved. Intravenous hydration continued for several hours after the transplant.

Harry was so worn out from that day; I am not sure if it was from the transplant or his stress level from turning that dial on and off. He was so serious about it and he was so hilarious for the rest of us to watch that we would not give that picture up for anything. They sedated Harry to let him rest well that evening. I, in turn, had met others on our transplant floor and would go visit. There was another couple about our age and he had the transplant and came through with flying colors. He was one of the patients that started his transplant from his first diagnosis of mantle cell and he had minimal complications. So you see we are not the only family that has or will ever go through this trying time, but maybe we can help many of you out there make an all important decision on a stem cell transplant and if it is right for you.

"Learn from yesterday, live for today, hope for tomorrow."

(Unkown)

21

Post Stem Cell Transplant

The next morning the hospital room was still bare of everything except my oh-so comfortable bed and Harry's oh-so comfortable hospital bed. Monitors were hooked to Harry as it takes time for the stem cells to be accepted and start working within the body. A serious complication set in as Harry's heartbeat accelerated and the cardiac team was brought in within minutes. They readied the electric paddles and I was so shocked because I knew they thought his heart might stop. A shot was administered to Harry and his heart slowed down and the paddles did not have to be used after all. He did have a mild heart attack but he was back on track. The cardiologist team explained to me that as fast as his heart was beating they would have stopped his heart and then started it back at the regular pace using the paddles. It is amazing everything that we have learned with this journey.

Each day that went by Harry was a bit stronger and was very coherent. Dr. Hurd, one of the senior doctors jokingly told Harry that one-day he observes a transplant, the next day he assists, and the third day he would perform one. That is their protocol motto so they thought Harry would like to join their team since he had spent so much time with them and assisted with the dial with his own transplant.

Harry started to give the nurses a hard time so they knew that he was back on the mend. He told Kathy, his nurse, that she could not remember to bring him his meds and she needed sticky notes. She played along so great that the next time she came into his room she had yellow sticky notes all over her so he could write his complaints down. He complained that he had no privacy when anyone came into the room so I used two IV poles and a hospital gown and made a privacy curtain for him. The curtain was in the shape of a horse and when it was up doctors and nurses alike knew that Harry was doing his business so do not come in at this time. The psychologist came into our room for our counseling session and he loved the idea of decorating and making ourselves feel at home so he took a picture of our horse divider. He would like to let other families know that there are others of us in the same place in life but you must keep your spirits up and continue with HOPE. He also believes that corporate America needs to know that the patients need the support of their immediate family member and many times this would make the difference in the patient living or dying during a transplant such as Harry and many others have gone through.

Harry was on an IV and antibiotics and was growing stronger each day. His skin color was very jaundice and his hair was gone again, but he was talking and still giving the nurses more hard times. He kept rubbing his blood type from his hospital bracelet and so Kathy once more came in with the best joke on him. She made small stickers and placed them on all of his toenails. You know he was back when he could dish it out and also take it. It was only eight days after the transplant and Harry was doing great for what he had just gone through.

I went home to sterilize the home with bleach and get it ready for a very immune deficient person to be able to survive in our surroundings. We purchased an air purifier with an ionize filter to keep the home air as pure as the hospital. That has been a great asset to our home. I spent all day Saturday and into the evening cleaning bathrooms, kitchen, and carpets and then I was ready to go pick him up for the great return. Sunday morning I drove 1 ½ hours to pick up the sick patient. Harry returned home and I, the spouse caregiver, had to return to my full time job on Monday.

Anything that Harry would need was placed by his bedside as all family members were either at work or school and he was not physically able to get out of bed. On Monday Harry called me at work and his nose would not stop bleeding. I rushed home and packed his nose with gauze and rushed him to the Winston- Salem Baptist Hospital. He needed platelet and blood transfusions, as the cells had not started to clot yet. We returned home at 5:00 am and I had to return to work on

Tuesday morning. We had been home a total of 24 hours and already complications began. I called our hometown oncologist and she consulted with our protocol team and arrangements were made to do the maintenance follow-up appointments at the Gaston Memorial Hospital.

"Hope is like a road in the country; there was never a road, but when many people walk on it, the road comes into existence."

(Lin Yutang)

22

Daily Transfusions, Shots
and Counseling

He would need transfusions at least every other day and sometimes every day, and the nurses in the blood transfusion out patient department got to know Harry on a personal basis and cheered him on to victory. I also was taught to administer shots to Harry on a daily basis to build up his system. The entire family started to visit the oncology counselor in Gastonia and our children even made their own appointments when they thought they needed a little help through a crisis that they did not want to bother mom or dad with. The nurses on the oncology floor loved to see Harry come to the hospital as he was such a great patient even when he was deathly sick or had pneumonia. We were informed that cancer would not be the culprit that finally killed Harry but pneumonia or something to do with his lungs as his lungs are now like shear glass.

Within a month Harry started to get stronger and the platelet transfusions stopped completely and he also did not need so many blood transfusions. He attended physical therapy treatment and an exercise program and slowly but surely he was coming back to full strength. When a stem cell transplant is received the whole realm of physical and mental therapy and exercise is very important, as the whole body has gone through a tremendous change. Harry has always told us that he would never be the same person that he once was because he had been to deaths door so many times. He learned to take each day, minute, and second at a time and to enjoy the small things in life. Big expensive things mean nothing if you do not have life and a loving family to enjoy them with. He slowed down in life and enjoyed that he was still alive.

"It's kind of fun to do the impossible."
(Unknown)

23

Remission

Just seven months later in June of 2003, Harry was well enough to go on a camping trip with teenagers from our church. He even slept in a tent on the ground although we did cheat and take a foam mattress to sleep on. We will let you in on a secret. If you have all of these problems with your lungs DO NOT dive into the deep end of a swimming pool. What a shock to Harry as he dove in and his lungs would not fill with air and he could not float. Someone had to actually jump in to save him from drowning and he said that was a very scary feeling.

Harry stayed well and even went back to work in 2003 for one year. Harry still went for monthly appointments to Winston-Salem so they could track his progress for the protocol study. We wrote articles for our hometown newspaper three years in a row and Harry was the speaker for Relay for Life for two years. He was such an inspiration for other cancer patients and many just wanted to shake his hand for being chosen from our small town to become part of such an awesome protocol team in the effort to research new avenues in the cancer field.

Remission lasted for almost three years to the day. He was lacking only four days of getting to his fourth birthday November 1, 2005.

"Good timber does not grow with ease.
The stronger the wind the stronger the trees."
(J. Willard Marriott)

24

Cancer Returns

In August of 2005, Harry called me at work at 10:00am and asked what time I was taking my lunch hour. I could tell that his words were slurred and immediately asked what was wrong. He said that he thought he had a stroke and was in bed. Of course I did not wait until lunch and I called a friend to help load him into the car to head for the emergency room. Sure enough, he was right. He had a TIA which is a small stroke that is usually a warning that a larger stroke may occur. He was in the hospital for some time, but he recovered very well and all went back to normal.

Then in October of 2005 he came down with double pneumonia and was placed in the hospital once more. He went for his PET scan and CAT scan and on October 27, 2005 it was discovered that his cancer had returned in his neck, stomach, and groin. This was just days before his three-year anniversary of remission. What a blow, but when we think about it, we cannot complain as we had Harry longer than we would have without a stem cell transplant. We had an opportunity to live a medical phenomenon and now I am able to write a book to let others know what to expect in the worse case scenario. We can say that we have lived one of the most interesting lives in America. All stem cell transplants are not complicated like Harry's, but all are not the express lane either.

"Courage is not defined by those who fought and did not fall, but by those who fought, fell and rose again."

(Unknown)

25

Possible Allo Stem Cell Transplant

Do Not Resuscitate

To continue with Harry's cancer journey, as you remember in the earlier part of this book, the doctor discussed the allo transplant (donor stem cells) if his sister was a match. We visited Winston-Salem Baptist Hospital immediately after the cancer had resurfaced in three areas of his body. Since Harry was first diagnosed our hometown oncologist had moved back to Tennessee to take a research position and we were very fortunate to have yet another excellent oncologist as our team captain. Dr. Matulis actually worked at Winston- Salem Baptist Hospital and we were introduced to her before we returned home from our long visits in the Baptist Hospital. We chose her and she chose us as one of her first patients in the Gaston region.

Harry was to begin eight sessions of week-long chemo treatments to get ready for a possible donor stem cell transplant. This chemo was different than the others. Harry would not get a two-week reprieve but only four days between each session and this would equate to forty chemo treatments. After just the first week of chemo, Harry was admitted into the hospital for seven days as the wicked, yet wonderful, drug chemo tried to claim his life. He was released from the hospital just to be admitted back within two days. Again, the entire hospital staff that worked with him gave him all the healing attention and moral support he could ever ask for. When he finally got out of the hospital, he had daily blood and platelet transfusions again and stood tough through it all.

Within four weeks Harry started his second session of chemo and this time it did almost claim his life. On November 30, 2005 we admitted Harry into emergency care just to learn that his entire system had shut down. We were told that he was at the end of life, and I, as the power of attorney, had to step in and have his lungs pressurized to keep him living. I knew my husband and I knew that he had fought too hard to go this far just to give up to a chemo malfunction. He did survive and made a miraculous recovery. Another thing that we learned during this test is what 'Do Not Resuscitate' really means to a patient and the power of attorney. Of course we had DNR paperwork drawn up by our attorney and we carried it with us each time we went to the hospital. When the time comes and you have to make the decision there is a big difference if your loved one has to be placed on a ventilator or if they can be revived. Be very careful if you have paperwork that says DNR because if the power of attorney is not in the presence the DNR will be recognized. Check with your team on the difference of Do Not Intibate and DNR.

One more trip to Winston-Salem to consult with Dr. Keung and Harry would start another new regime of intravenous antibiotic/chemo to either maintain or even hopefully shrink the cancer cells. He received the last of his eight treatments and was on the verge of pneumonia for five weeks. After three z-packs for pneumonia and numerous other prescriptions, he got through with flying colors.

After the chemo treatment was complete there was a PET scan one more time to show that the areas of cancer had either shrunk or at least stayed the same. Harry found out that he would not be able to receive an allo transplant, as his system would not make it through anything of such magnitude. He did go through radiation on his neck to stop any further growth of this area. This is referred to 'spot welding'. Harry also went through a new complication of his blood pressure dropping when he stood up and this made him pass out and fall, which is very dangerous for broken bones. We were dealing with that and trying to find a remedy. In the meantime, his immune system was building and he was getting ready to receive yet another regime of intravenous antibiotic/chemo for the two small cancerous nodes remaining in his stomach.

"Courage is like love, it must have hope for nourishment."
(Napoleon I)

<u>26</u>

We are Still Hanging in There

The amazing thing is Harry started this journey of cancer February of 2001 and the best part of this story is he is still right here beside me as I write this book for him going on seven years later. Is a stem cell transplant right for you? It gave us **<u>HOPE</u>** but we are only one family of many who have to make the decision. Good Luck with your all so important decision.

I had a beautiful cousin, Missie, from Michigan that had a stem cell transplant two years before Harry and it prolonged her life by years. She has since passed on but she will always be a beautiful part of our life and she was such an inspiration to us for our decision in the stem cell transplant research study protocol.

<u>27</u>

Goodbye

Harry passed away in 2008 but not without a tremendous fight. Of course as the doctors predicted it was not the actual cancer, but kidney failure that claimed his life.

Before he left this earth he encouraged me to attend college to pursue my nursing degree. I enrolled into Gaston College January of 2008 and he passed away March of that year.

I have been accepted into the nursing program and will fulfill <u>our</u> last dream together.

"A hero is one who knows how to hang on one minute longer."

(Norwegian Proverb)

If you never try you will never know.

Fear is a thief of dreams.

There are almost 1,000 hospitals throughout the country that are performing bone marrow and stem cell transplants on cancer patients with great success!

Cancer is not the KISS OF DEATH.

"Life is very simple: it merely consists in learning how to accept the impossible, how to do without the indispensable, and how to endure the insupportable."
(Kathleen Norris)

"Every time you meet a situation, though you think at the time it is an impossibility and you go through the tortures of the damned, once you have met it and lived through it, you find that forever after you are freer than you were before."
(Eleanor Roosevelt)

Have you ever wondered what a stem cell transplant would really be like? We hope this will help you in your transplant decision. Would we go through it again? The answer is YES, and with all of the research that has been completed since our experience; it can only be better.

The staff at Mayo Clinic defines a stem cell transplant as the infusion of healthy stem cells into your body.

Although the procedure to replenish your body's supply of healthy blood-forming cells is generally called a stem cell transplant, it's also known as a bone marrow transplant or an umbilical cord blood transplant, depending on the source of the stem cells. Stem cell transplants can use cells from your own body (autologous stem cell transplant) or they can utilize stem cells from donors (allogenic stem cell transplant).

A special THANKS to my beloved husband.

Thank you for such an interesting life journey and making our family realize what life is about and what is really important.

On Harry's last trip to the emergency room he said, "I cannot go before the book is complete because my wife cannot get all of the glory."

I replied, "Babe, I will get none of the glory as I am now on page 69, if I were living the story instead of telling it I would have never made it past page 19."

You are our Hero

With All My Love

"Self-esteem must be earned! When you dare to dream, dare to suffer through the pain, sacrifice, self-doubt, and friction from the world, you will genuinely impress yourself."
(Laura Schiessinger)

Sandy Holmes now resides in Gastonia, North Carolina in the home that Harry bought her with his dying wish. She will finish Nursing School in mid 2012.

www.ingramcontent.com/pod-product-compliance
Lightning Source LLC
Chambersburg PA
CBHW022100170526
45157CB00004B/1418